Choosing Eyeglasses with Mrs. Koutris

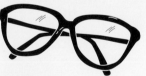

written by
ALICE K. FLANAGAN

photographs by
ROMIE FLANAGAN

Reading Consultant
LINDA CORNWELL
Learning Resource Consultant
Indiana Department of Education

CHILDREN'S PRESS®   *A Division of Grolier Publishing*
New York • London • Hong Kong • Sydney • Danbury, Connecticut

Special thanks to Linda Koutris for allowing us to tell her story.

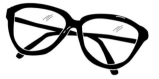

Also, thanks to Dr. May and Deerfield Optical.

Author's Note:

Mrs. Koutris's last name is pronounced KOOTRIS.

Library of Congress Cataloging-in-Publication Data

Flanagan, Alice.

    Choosing eyeglasses with Mrs. Koutris / written by Alice K. Flanagan ; photographs by Romie Flanagan.

       p.   cm. — (Our neighborhood)

    Summary: Follows an optician as she helps her customers find glasses that suit them and let them see better.

    ISBN 0-516-20775-X (lib. bdg.)   0-516-26294-7 (pbk.)

    1. Opticianry—Juvenile literature. 2. Eyeglasses—Juvenile literature. [1. Opticians. 2. Eyeglasses. 3. Occupations.] I. Flanagan, Romie, ill. II. Title. III. Series: Our neighborhood (New York, N.Y.)

    RE952.F57   1998

    617.7'522—dc21

                                   97-11864

                                       CIP

                                       AC

Photographs ©: Romie Flanagan

      7 8 9 10 R 10 09 08

                      62

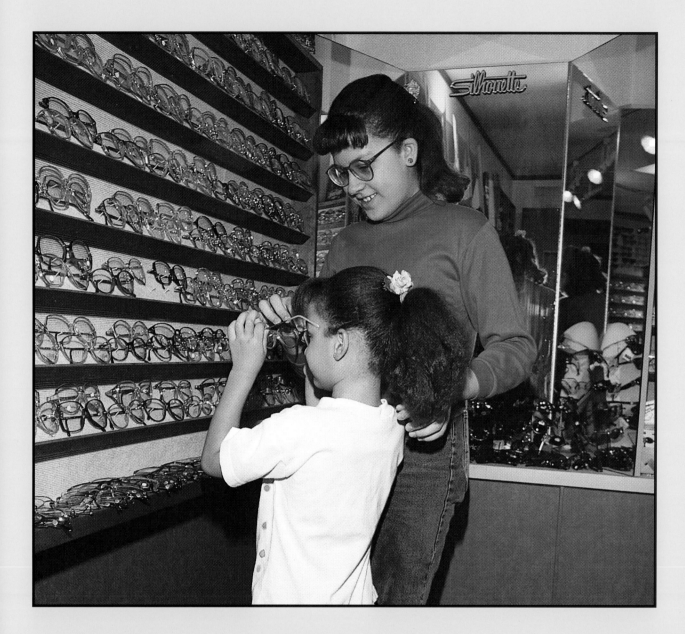

If you need eyeglasses, Mrs. Koutris's office is the place to go.

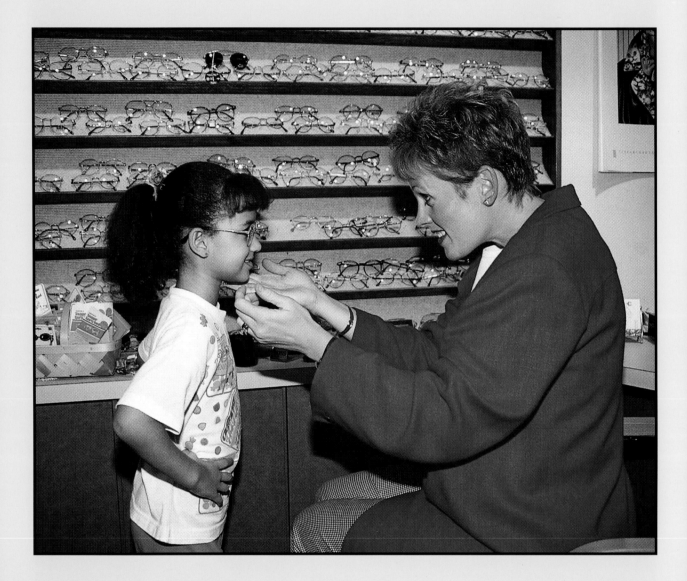

There are hundreds of colorful frames to choose from.

Mrs. Koutris
will help you
find a pair that
fits just right!

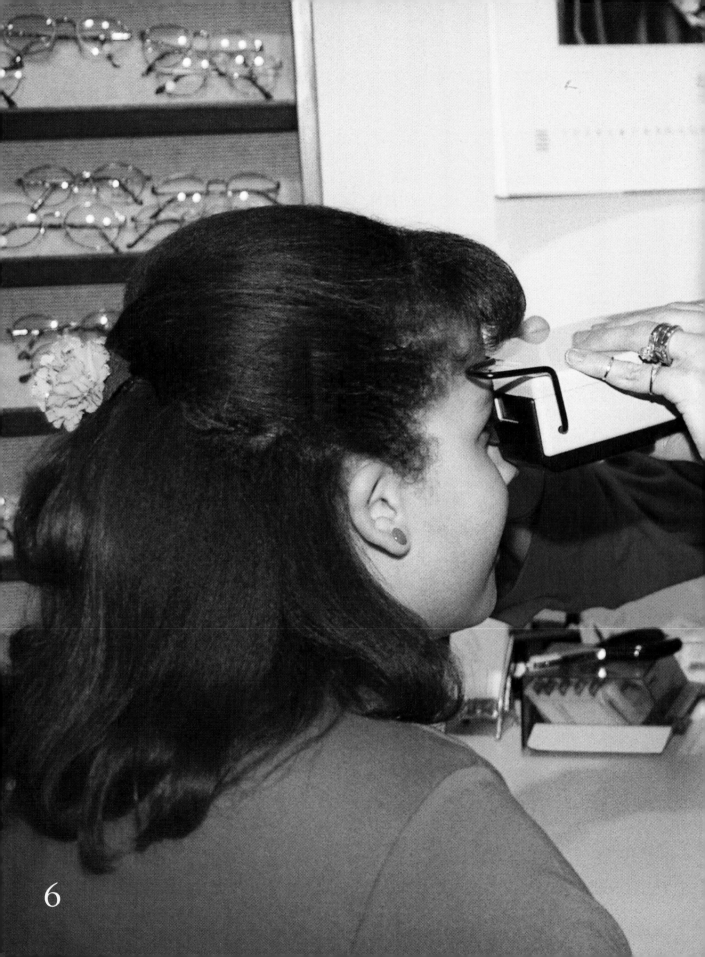

Mrs. Koutris is an optician.
She helps people see better.

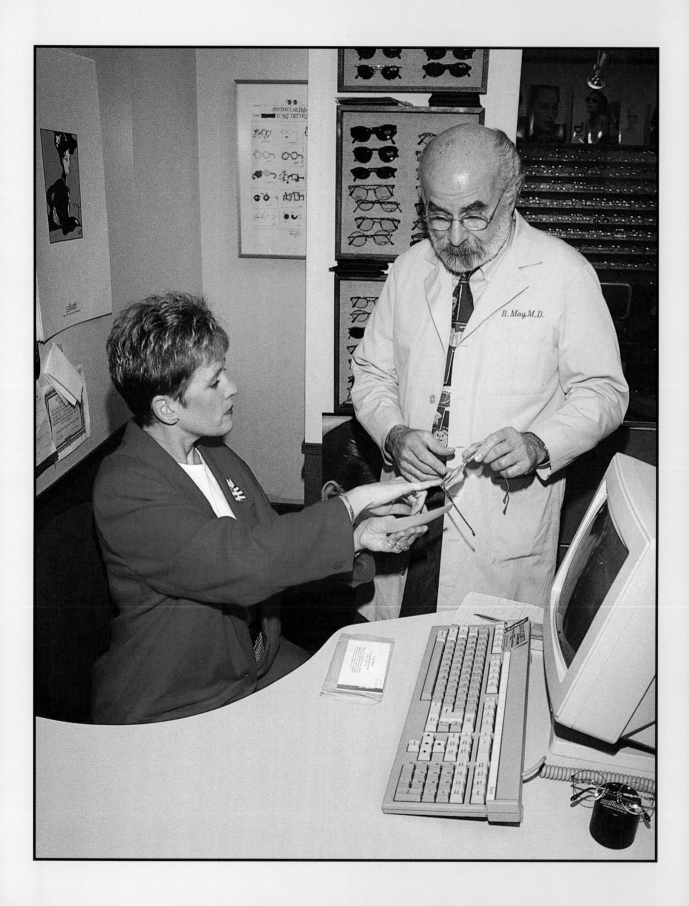

She works closely with Dr. May.
He examines the patients' eyes and
writes down what kind of lenses
they need.

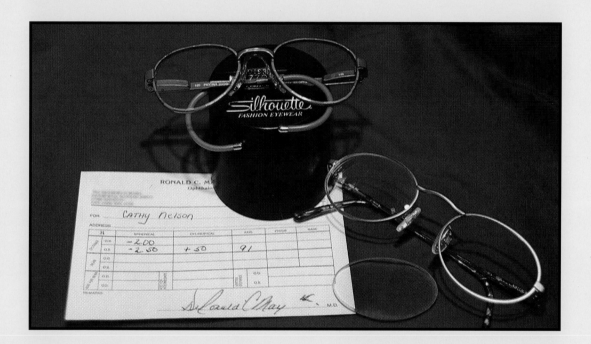

Dr. May's order is called
a prescription.

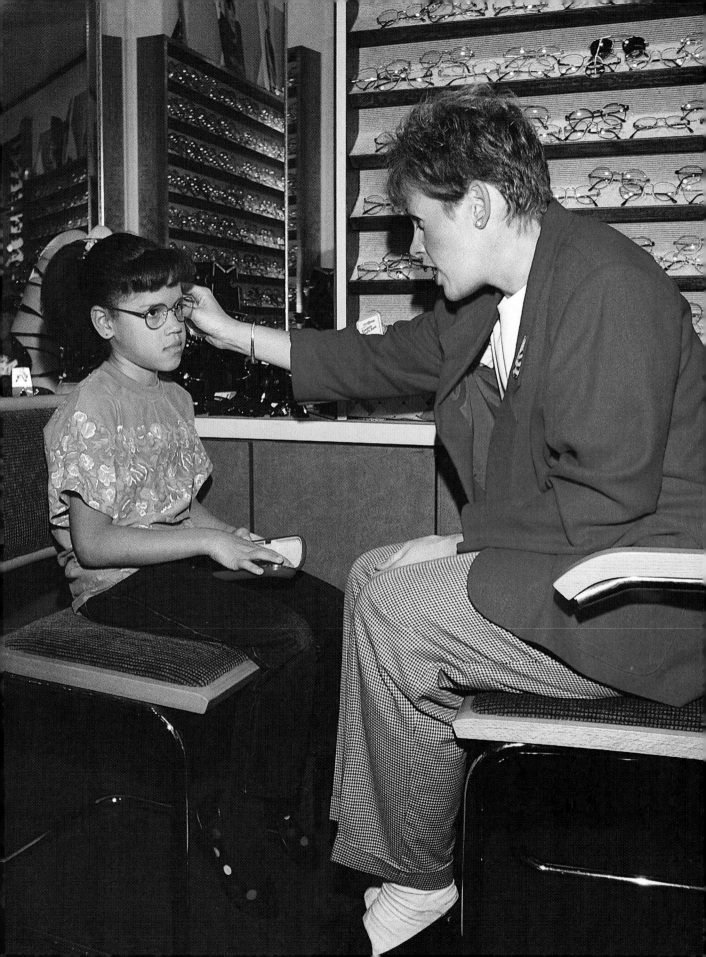

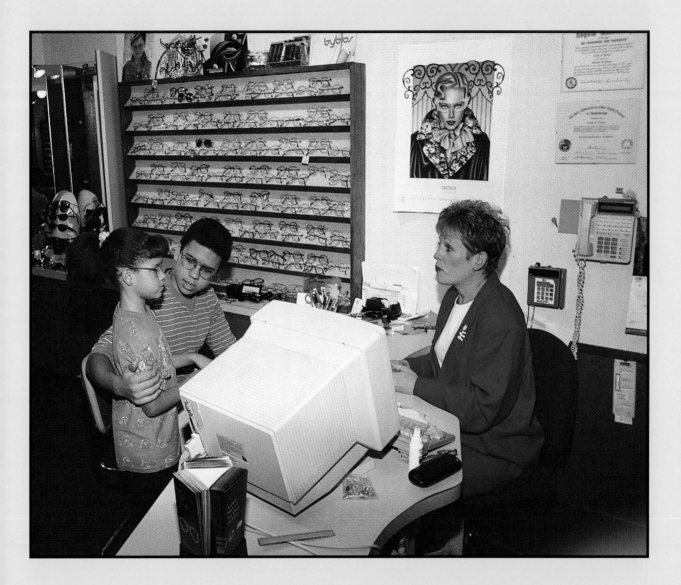

Mrs. Koutris helps patients pick frames that look good on their faces.

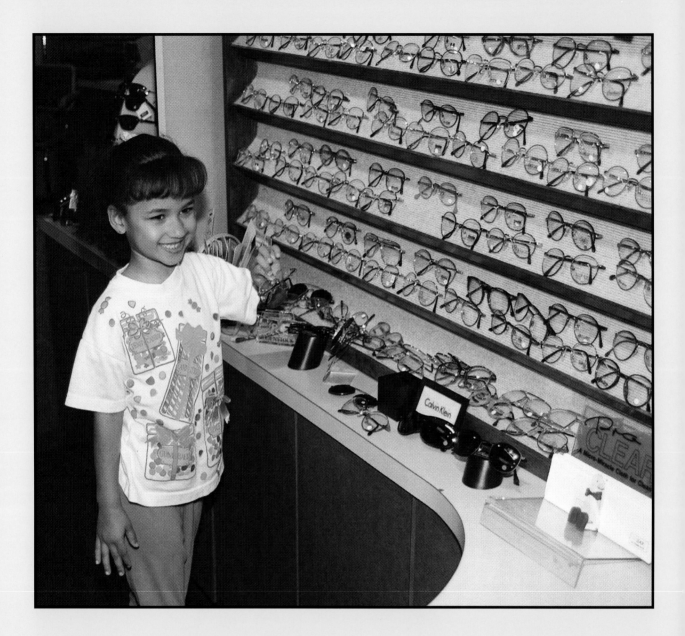

Often, people choose frames that
are their favorite color.

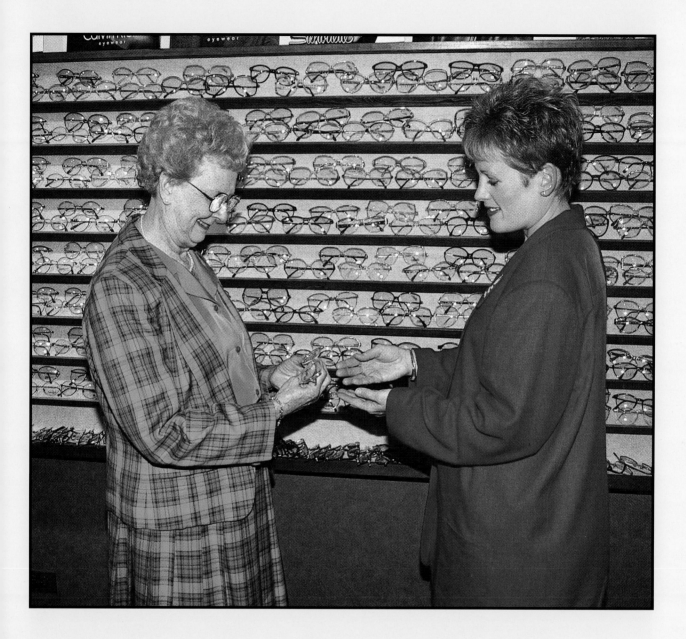

Sometimes, they pick ones that are a certain shape.

Sports frames should fit nice
and tight so they don't fall off
during a game.

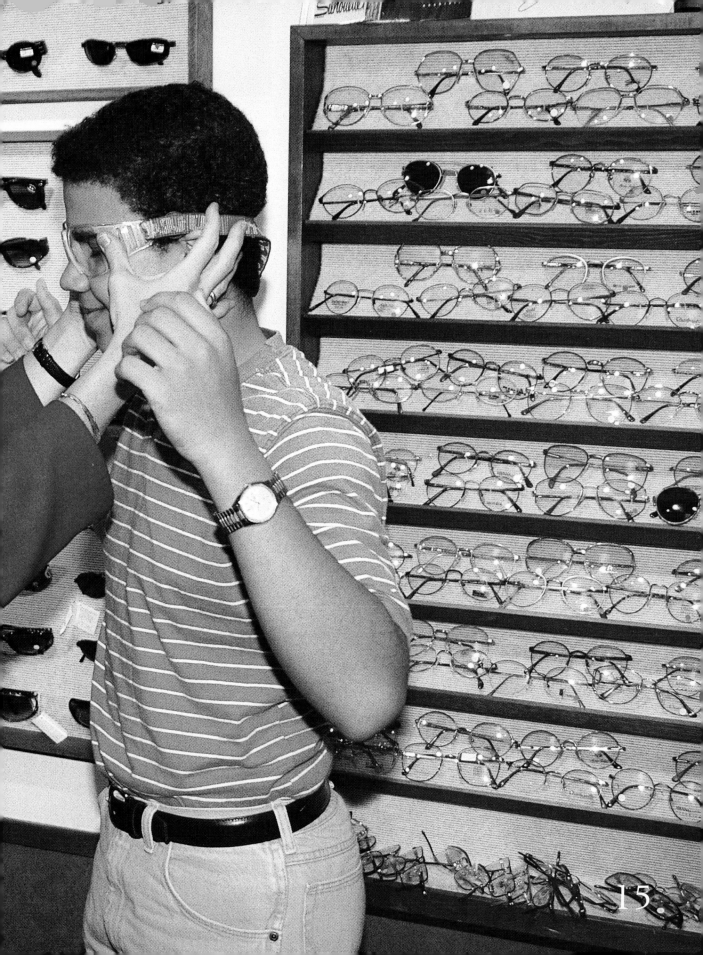

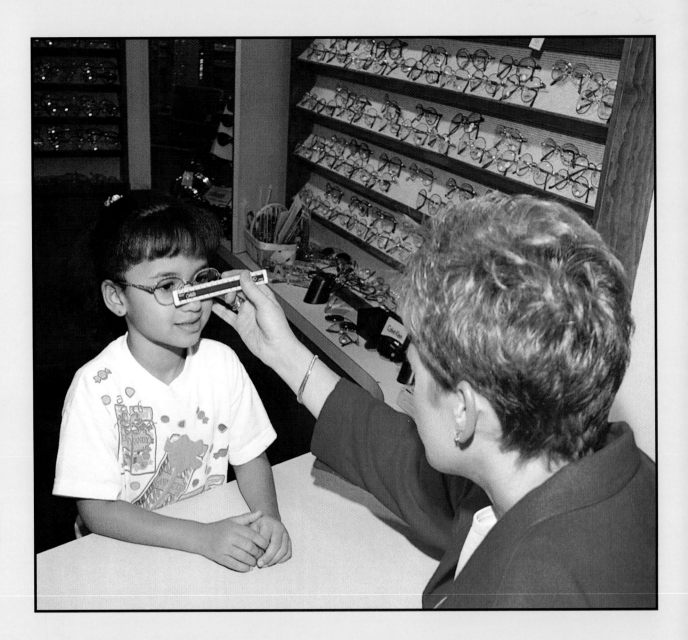

Mrs. Koutris measures the space
between the patient's eyes. She
writes down the information.

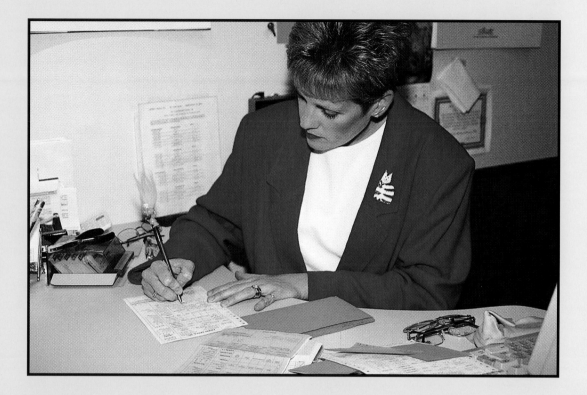

Then, she sends this information with the prescription and the frames to the lens makers. They make the lenses and place them into the frames.

Soon, the glasses
come back from the
lens makers.

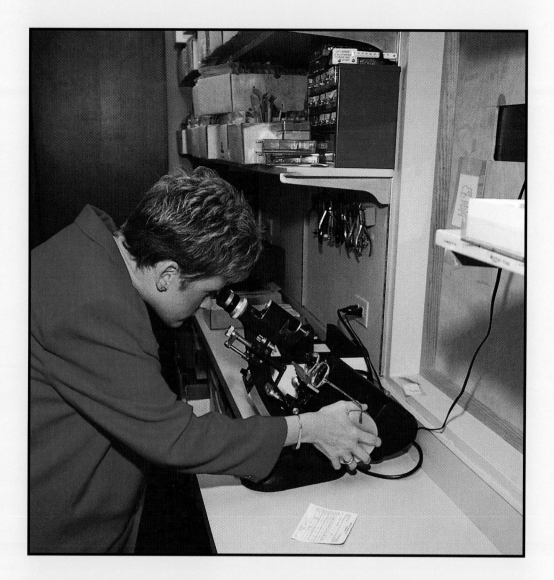

Mrs. Koutris tests the lenses to see
if they are correct.

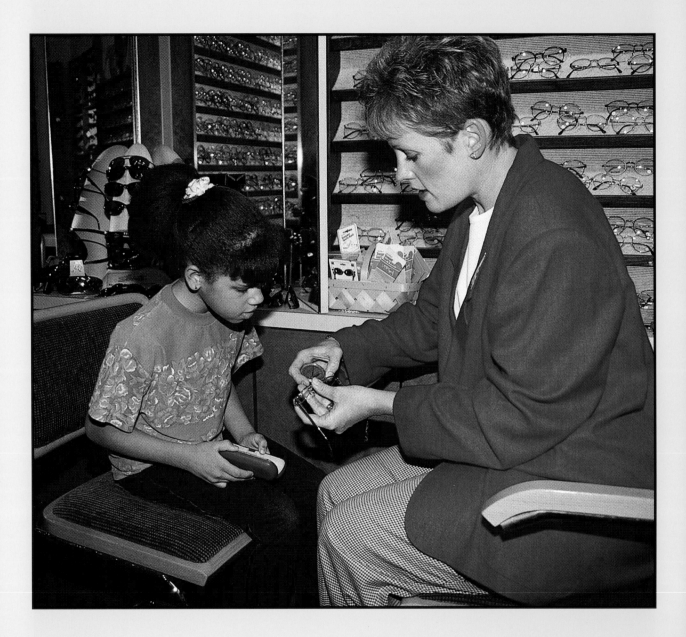

Are they what the doctor ordered?

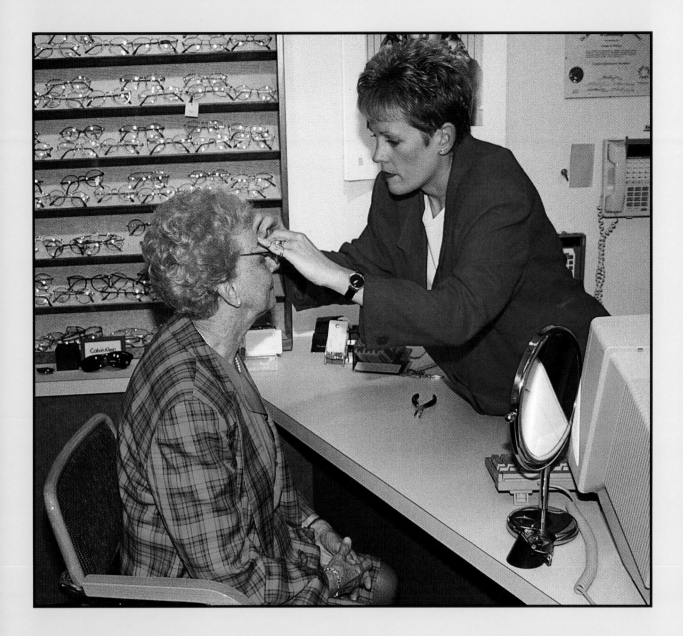

Do they fit in the frames?

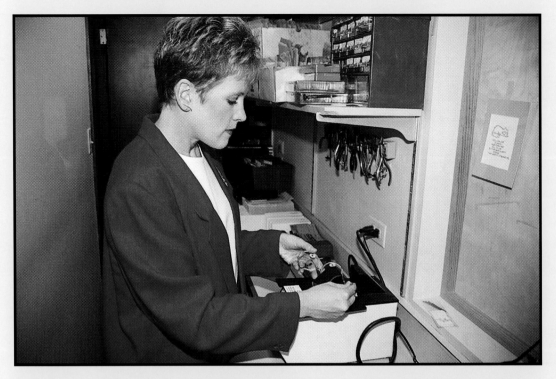

Sometimes, she heats the frames

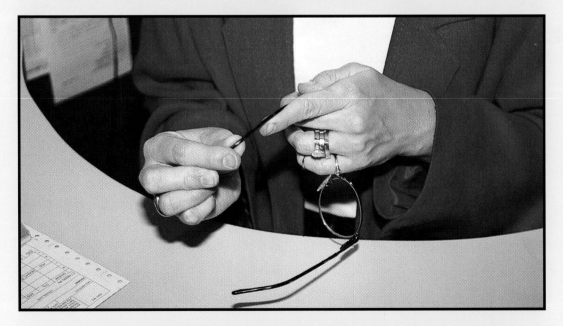

so they can be bent and shaped.

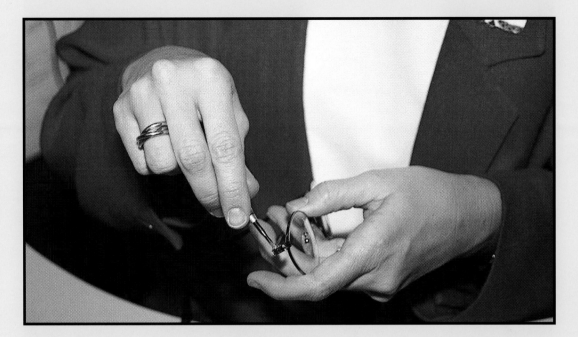

Finally, she tightens loose parts with a screwdriver

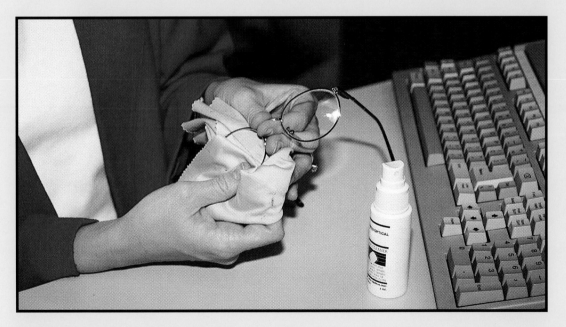

and cleans the lenses well.

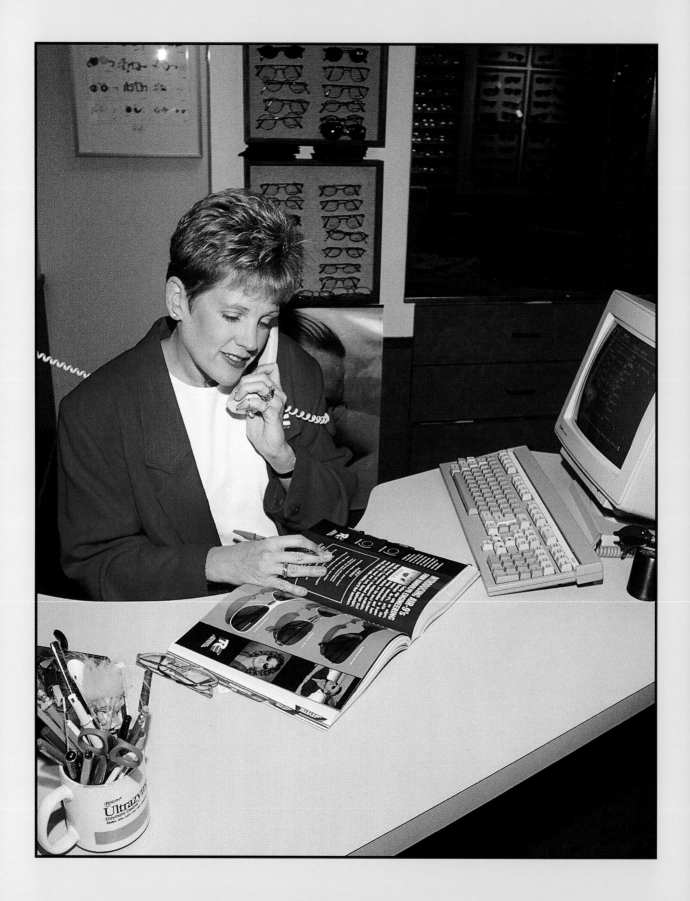

When Mrs. Koutris is not with a patient, she orders supplies

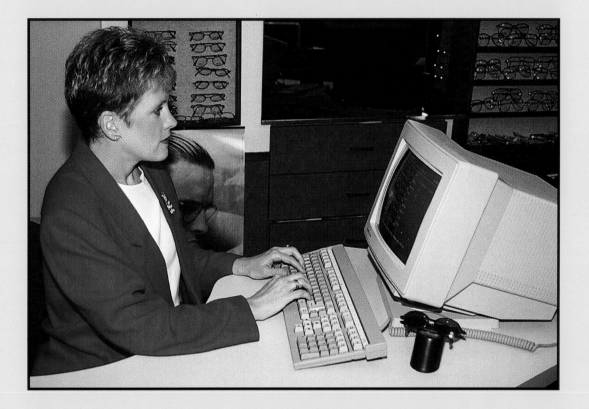

and types information into the computer.

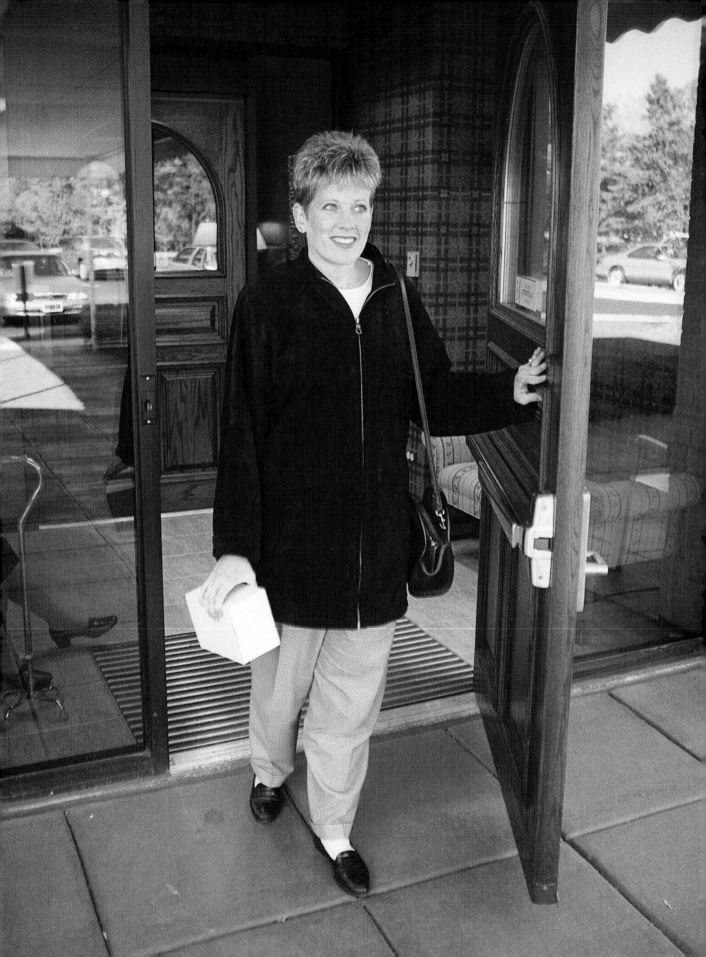

Sometimes, sick or older patients can't pick up their eyeglasses at Mrs. Koutris's office. So Mrs. Koutris brings the eyeglasses to them.

Meeting people is what Mrs. Koutris likes most about her job. She listens carefully to what patients want and helps choose the best eyeglasses for them.

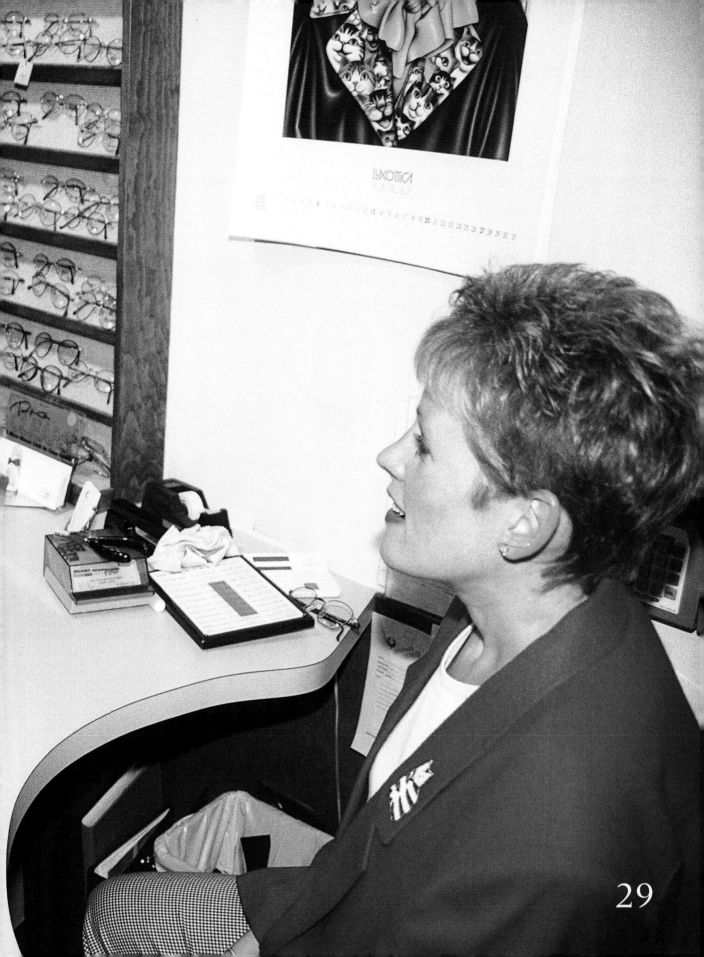

29

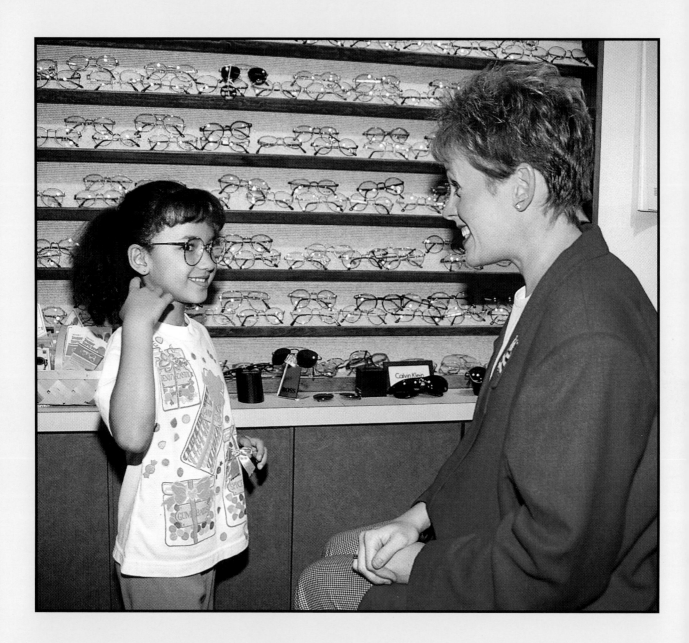

People are happy when they leave
Mrs. Koutris's office.

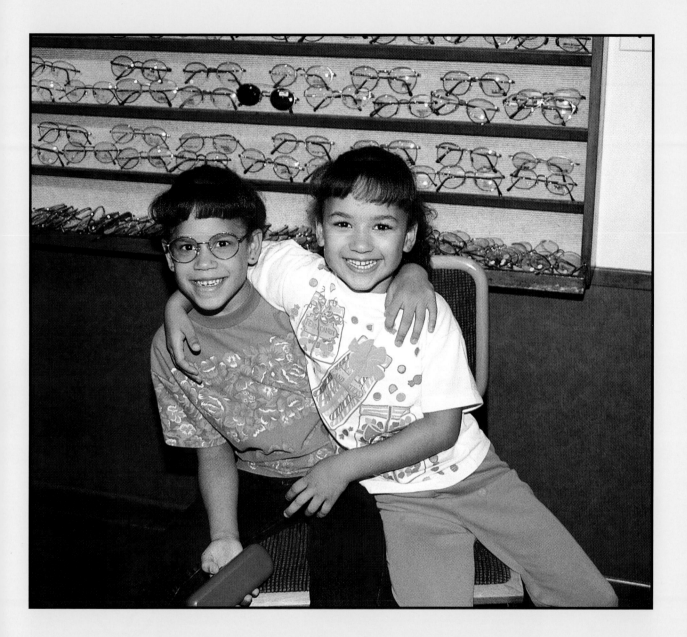

Because of her help, they can see
everything in the world better
than before!

Meet the Author
and the Photographer

Alice and Romie Flanagan live in Chicago, Illinois, and have been involved in bookmaking for many years. Alice is a writer, and Romie is a photographer. As husband and wife, they enjoy working together closely. They hope their books help children learn about the people in their community and how their jobs affect their neighborhood.

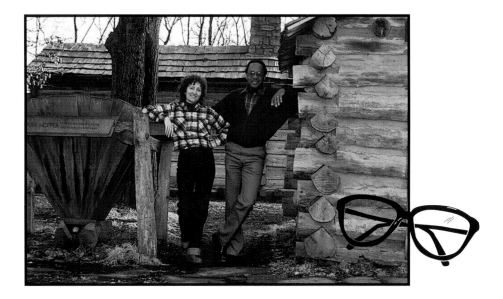